THE CONSTIPATION DIET BIBLE

Nutritional Solutions For Constipation And A Dietary Guide To Easier Digestive Health

CRUE GAGE

Copyright © 2024 By Crue Gage

All Rights Reserved.

Table of Contents

Introductory 4

CHAPTER ONE 8

  How The Digestive System Works & Factors Affecting Digestion 8

  Symptoms And Causes 12

  Foods To Avoid & Foods To Include 15

CHAPTER TWO 19

  7 Days Sample Meal Plans 19

  Breakfast Recipes 25

  Lunch Recipes 30

  Dinner Recipes 36

  Snacks & Desserts Recipes 43

CHAPTER THREE 49

  Supplements And Natural Remedies 49

  Lifestyle Factors 53

  Monitoring And Adjusting Your Diet 55

  Conclusion 59

THE END 61

Introductory

Constipation is a common digestive issue characterized by infrequent bowel movements or difficulty passing stools. It can lead to hard, dry stools that are painful to pass.

Symptoms May Include:

- Infrequent bowel movements (typically fewer than three times a week)
- Straining during bowel movements
- A feeling of incomplete evacuation
- Abdominal discomfort or bloating

Causes of constipation can vary and may include a low-fiber diet, dehydration, lack of physical activity, certain medications, or underlying health conditions. Treatment often involves lifestyle changes, such as increasing fiber intake, drinking more water, and exercising regularly. In some cases, over-the-counter laxatives may be recommended.

Diet plays a crucial role in managing constipation. Here are key ways in which dietary choices can help alleviate and prevent this condition:

• **Fiber Intake**: Consuming a diet high in fiber can promote regular bowel movements. Soluble fiber (found in oats, beans, and fruits) helps soften stools, while insoluble fiber (found in whole grains, nuts, and vegetables) adds bulk and aids movement through the digestive tract.

• **Hydration**: Drinking plenty of water is essential, as adequate hydration helps soften stool, making it easier to pass. Aim for at least eight glasses a day, or more if you're physically active.

- **Fruits and Vegetables**: Incorporating a variety of fruits and vegetables not only increases fiber intake but also provides important nutrients. Fruits like prunes, apples, and pears are particularly helpful due to their natural sugars and fiber.

- **Whole Grains**: Whole grains, such as brown rice, whole wheat bread, and quinoa, are rich in fiber and can contribute to improved digestive health.

- **Limit Processed Foods**: Reducing the intake of processed and high-fat foods can help, as they often lack fiber and can contribute to constipation.

- **Regular Meals**: Eating regular meals and snacks can stimulate the digestive system and promote more regular bowel movements.

- **Probiotics**: Foods that contain probiotics, such as yogurt and fermented foods, can help maintain a healthy gut flora, which is beneficial for digestion.

By making these dietary adjustments, individuals can often reduce the frequency and severity of constipation episodes.

CHAPTER ONE
How The Digestive System Works & Factors Affecting Digestion

The digestive system is responsible for breaking down food, absorbing nutrients, and eliminating waste. Here's a brief overview of how it works and factors that can affect digestion:

How the Digestive System Works:

- **Mouth**: Digestion begins here, where food is mechanically broken down by chewing and mixed with saliva, which contains enzymes that start the digestion of carbohydrates.

- **Esophagus**: Swallowed food travels down the esophagus via muscular contractions called peristalsis, reaching the stomach.

- **Stomach**: Food is mixed with gastric juices, which contain acid and enzymes that further break down proteins. The stomach churns food into a semi-liquid substance called chyme.

- **Small Intestine**: Chyme moves into the small intestine, where most nutrient absorption occurs. The pancreas releases digestive enzymes, and the liver produces bile (stored in the gallbladder) to help digest fats.

- **Large Intestine**: Undigested food moves into the large intestine, where water and electrolytes are absorbed. The remaining waste is formed into stool.

- **Rectum and Anus**: Stool is stored in the rectum until it is expelled through the anus during a bowel movement.

Factors Affecting Digestion:

- **Diet**: High-fat or low-fiber diets can slow digestion, while fiber-rich foods promote regularity.

- **Hydration**: Adequate water intake is crucial for softening stool and facilitating movement through the digestive tract.

- **Physical Activity**: Regular exercise promotes gut motility, aiding digestion and preventing constipation.

- **Stress**: High-stress levels can disrupt the digestive process, potentially leading to issues like indigestion, bloating, or diarrhea.

- **Medications**: Some medications, such as certain pain relievers, antidepressants, and iron supplements, can affect digestion and may lead to constipation or diarrhea.

- **Health Conditions**: Conditions like irritable bowel syndrome (IBS), diabetes, hypothyroidism, or gastrointestinal disorders can significantly impact digestive health.

- **Aging**: The digestive system may slow down with age, leading to issues like constipation.

Understanding these factors can help individuals make informed choices to support their digestive health.

Symptoms And Causes

Symptoms of Constipation:

- **Infrequent Bowel Movements**: Fewer than three times a week.
- **Straining**: Difficulty or pain when trying to pass stools.
- **Hard or Lumpy Stools**: Stools that are dry and difficult to pass.
- **Abdominal Discomfort**: Bloating, cramping, or pain in the abdomen.
- **Feeling of Incomplete Evacuation**: The sensation that the bowels have not completely emptied.

Causes of Constipation:

Dietary Factors:

- Low fiber intake (fruits, vegetables, whole grains).

- Insufficient fluid intake.

Lifestyle Factors:

- Lack of physical activity.
- Ignoring the urge to have a bowel movement.

Medications:

- Pain medications (especially opioids).
- Antidepressants and certain antacids.
- Iron supplements.

Health Conditions:

- Irritable bowel syndrome (IBS).
- Hypothyroidism.
- Diabetes.

- Neurological disorders (e.g., Parkinson's disease, multiple sclerosis).

Hormonal Changes: Hormonal fluctuations during pregnancy or menopause can affect digestion.

- **Aging**: Digestive processes may slow down with age.

- **Stress and Anxiety**: Emotional stress can impact gut function and lead to constipation.

Understanding these symptoms and causes can help in identifying and addressing constipation effectively.

Foods To Avoid & Foods To Include

Foods to Avoid for Constipation:

Low-Fiber Foods:

- White bread and pasta
- Processed cereals
- Snack foods (chips, crackers)

Dairy Products:

- Cheese and full-fat dairy (can be binding for some people)

Red Meat:

- High in fat and low in fiber.

Fried and Fast Foods:

- High in unhealthy fats and low in fiber.

Processed Foods:

- Foods with added sugars and preservatives.

Caffeinated Beverages:

- Excessive caffeine can lead to dehydration.

Alcohol:

- Can be dehydrating, leading to constipation.

<u>Foods to Include for Healthy Digestion:</u>

High-Fiber Foods:

- Whole grains (brown rice, quinoa, whole wheat bread)
- Beans and legumes (lentils, chickpeas, black beans)

- Fruits (apples, pears, berries, prunes)
- Vegetables (broccoli, carrots, leafy greens)

Hydrating Foods:

• Cucumbers, watermelon, oranges, and other water-rich fruits and vegetables.

Probiotic Foods:

• Yogurt, kefir, sauerkraut, kimchi, and other fermented foods to support gut health.

Nuts and Seeds:

• Almonds, chia seeds, and flaxseeds are good sources of fiber and healthy fats.

Healthy Fats:

- Olive oil, avocados, and fatty fish can support digestion.

Adequate Fluids:

- Water, herbal teas, and broths help keep stools soft.

Incorporating high-fiber foods and staying hydrated can significantly improve digestive health and help prevent constipation.

CHAPTER TWO
7 Days Sample Meal Plans

Here's a 7-day sample meal plan to help manage constipation, focusing on high-fiber foods, hydration, and balanced nutrition.

Day 1:

- **Breakfast**: Overnight oats with chia seeds, topped with berries and a drizzle of honey.
- **Snack**: An apple with almond butter.
- **Lunch**: Quinoa salad with black beans, corn, diced bell peppers, and a lime vinaigrette.
- **Snack**: Carrot sticks and hummus.
- **Dinner**: Grilled salmon with steamed broccoli and brown rice.

Day 2:

- **Breakfast**: Whole grain toast with avocado and a poached egg.
- **Snack**: Greek yogurt with sliced bananas and flaxseeds.
- **Lunch**: Lentil soup with a side of whole grain bread.
- **Snack**: Celery sticks with peanut butter.
- **Dinner**: Stir-fried tofu with mixed vegetables (bell peppers, broccoli, and snap peas) served with quinoa.

Day 3:

- **Breakfast**: Smoothie with spinach, banana, yogurt, and a tablespoon of chia seeds.
- **Snack**: A pear.

- **Lunch**: Spinach salad with chickpeas, cherry tomatoes, cucumbers, and balsamic dressing.
- **Snack**: Trail mix (nuts and dried fruits).
- **Dinner**: Whole wheat pasta with marinara sauce and sautéed vegetables.

Day 4:

- **Breakfast**: Oatmeal topped with sliced apples and cinnamon.
- **Snack**: A handful of almonds.
- **Lunch**: Brown rice bowl with black beans, avocado, salsa, and corn.
- **Snack**: Sliced bell peppers with guacamole.
- **Dinner**: Baked chicken breast with sweet potato and green beans.

Day 5:

- **Breakfast**: Whole grain pancakes topped with fresh berries and a bit of maple syrup.
- **Snack**: Orange slices.
- **Lunch**: Mixed bean salad with diced tomatoes, onions, and parsley.
- **Snack**: Greek yogurt with honey and walnuts.
- **Dinner**: Grilled shrimp with a side of quinoa and steamed asparagus.

Day 6:

- **Breakfast**: Smoothie bowl with blended bananas, spinach, and almond milk, topped with granola and seeds.
- **Snack**: Baby carrots with hummus.

- **Lunch**: Barley salad with roasted vegetables and feta cheese.
- **Snack**: An apple with cottage cheese.
- **Dinner**: Stuffed bell peppers with ground turkey, brown rice, and diced tomatoes.

Day 7:

- **Breakfast**: Chia pudding made with almond milk, topped with kiwi and coconut flakes.
- **Snack**: A handful of mixed nuts.
- **Lunch**: Whole grain wrap with turkey, spinach, and avocado.
- **Snack**: Sliced cucumbers with tzatziki sauce.
- **Dinner**: Grilled vegetable and chickpea stir-fry served with quinoa.

Tips:

- Stay hydrated throughout the day by drinking plenty of water.
- Adjust portion sizes according to your needs and preferences.
- Feel free to mix and match meals based on your taste and available ingredients.

Breakfast Recipes

Here are some delicious and fiber-rich breakfast recipes to help with digestion:

1. Overnight Oats:

Ingredients:

- 1/2 cup rolled oats
- 1 cup almond milk (or any milk of choice)
- 1 tablespoon chia seeds
- 1 tablespoon honey or maple syrup
- Toppings: berries, sliced banana, nuts

Instructions:

- In a jar or bowl, combine oats, almond milk, chia seeds, and sweetener.

- Stir well and refrigerate overnight.
- In the morning, add your favorite toppings before serving.

2. Avocado Toast:

Ingredients:

- 1 slice whole grain bread
- 1/2 ripe avocado
- Salt and pepper to taste
- Optional toppings: sliced tomatoes, radishes, poached egg, or red pepper flakes

Instructions:

- Toast the whole grain bread.
- Mash the avocado in a bowl and season with salt and pepper.
- Spread the mashed avocado on the toast and add any additional toppings.

3. Smoothie Bowl:

Ingredients:

- 1 banana
- 1 cup spinach
- 1/2 cup Greek yogurt
- 1/2 cup almond milk
- Toppings: granola, seeds, sliced fruit, coconut flakes

Instructions:

- Blend banana, spinach, Greek yogurt, and almond milk until smooth.
- Pour the smoothie into a bowl and top with granola, seeds, and fruit.

4. Chia Seed Pudding:

Ingredients:

- 1/4 cup chia seeds

- 1 cup almond milk (or any milk)
- 1 tablespoon maple syrup or honey
- Toppings: fresh fruit, nuts, or granola

Instructions:

- In a bowl, mix chia seeds, almond milk, and sweetener.
- Stir well and let it sit for 10 minutes, then stir again to avoid clumping.
- Refrigerate for at least 2 hours or overnight.
- Serve with your choice of toppings.

5. Whole Grain Pancakes:

Ingredients:

- 1 cup whole wheat flour
- 1 tablespoon baking powder

- 1 tablespoon sugar (optional)
- 1 cup almond milk (or any milk)
- 1 egg
- 1 tablespoon melted coconut oil or butter
- Toppings: fresh berries, maple syrup

Instructions:

- In a bowl, mix flour, baking powder, and sugar.
- In another bowl, whisk almond milk, egg, and melted oil.
- Combine wet and dry ingredients and stir until just mixed.
- Heat a non-stick skillet over medium heat and pour in batter to form pancakes.
- Cook until bubbles form, then flip and cook until golden brown.

- Serve with berries and maple syrup.

These recipes are not only delicious but also packed with nutrients and fiber to support digestive health!

Lunch Recipes

Here are some healthy and fiber-rich lunch recipes:

1. Quinoa Salad with Black Beans

Ingredients:

- 1 cup cooked quinoa
- 1 can black beans (rinsed and drained)
- 1 cup diced bell peppers
- 1/2 cup corn (fresh or frozen)
- 1/4 cup chopped cilantro
- Juice of 1 lime

- Salt and pepper to taste

Instructions:

- In a large bowl, combine quinoa, black beans, bell peppers, corn, and cilantro.
- Drizzle with lime juice and season with salt and pepper.
- Toss gently and serve chilled or at room temperature.

2. Lentil Soup:

Ingredients:

- 1 cup lentils (green or brown), rinsed
- 1 onion, chopped
- 2 carrots, diced
- 2 celery stalks, diced
- 3 garlic cloves, minced
- 6 cups vegetable broth

- 1 can diced tomatoes
- 1 teaspoon cumin
- Salt and pepper to taste

Instructions:

- In a large pot, sauté onion, carrots, and celery in a little olive oil until softened.
- Add garlic and sauté for another minute.
- Stir in lentils, vegetable broth, diced tomatoes, cumin, salt, and pepper.
- Bring to a boil, then reduce heat and simmer for 25-30 minutes or until lentils are tender.

<u>3. Spinach and Chickpea Salad:</u>

Ingredients:

- 4 cups fresh spinach

- 1 can chickpeas (rinsed and drained)
- 1/2 cup cherry tomatoes, halved
- 1/4 cup red onion, thinly sliced
- 1/4 cup feta cheese (optional)
- Dressing: olive oil, lemon juice, salt, and pepper

Instructions:

- In a large bowl, combine spinach, chickpeas, cherry tomatoes, red onion, and feta.
- Drizzle with olive oil and lemon juice, then season with salt and pepper.
- Toss gently and serve.

4. Stuffed Bell Peppers:

Ingredients:

- 2 large bell peppers (any color)

- 1 cup cooked brown rice or quinoa
- 1 can diced tomatoes
- 1/2 cup black beans (rinsed and drained)
- 1 teaspoon chili powder
- Salt and pepper to taste

Instructions:

- Preheat the oven to 375°F (190°C).
- Cut the tops off the bell peppers and remove seeds.
- In a bowl, mix rice or quinoa, diced tomatoes, black beans, chili powder, salt, and pepper.
- Stuff the mixture into the bell peppers and place them in a baking dish.
- Bake for 25-30 minutes until the peppers are tender.

5. Whole Wheat Wrap:

Ingredients:

- 1 whole wheat wrap
- 3-4 slices turkey or chicken breast
- 1/4 avocado, sliced
- Handful of spinach or mixed greens
- Sliced cucumbers and tomatoes
- Dressing: mustard, hummus, or yogurt

Instructions:

- Spread your chosen dressing on the wrap.
- Layer turkey or chicken, avocado, spinach, cucumbers, and tomatoes.
- Roll the wrap tightly, slice in half, and enjoy!

- These lunch recipes are nutritious, easy to prepare, and perfect for maintaining digestive health!

Dinner Recipes

Here are some delicious and healthy dinner recipes that are rich in fiber and nutrients:

1. Grilled Salmon with Steamed Broccoli and Brown Rice:

Ingredients:

- 2 salmon fillets
- Olive oil
- Salt and pepper
- Lemon wedges
- 2 cups broccoli florets
- 1 cup cooked brown rice

Instructions:

- Preheat the grill or a grill pan over medium heat.
- Brush salmon fillets with olive oil and season with salt and pepper.
- Grill salmon for about 4-5 minutes on each side, or until cooked through.
- Steam broccoli until tender (about 5-7 minutes).
- Serve salmon with broccoli and brown rice, garnished with lemon wedges.

2. Stir-Fried Tofu and Mixed Vegetables:

Ingredients:

- 1 block firm tofu, drained and cubed

- 2 cups mixed vegetables (bell peppers, carrots, snap peas, etc.)
- 2 tablespoons soy sauce
- 1 tablespoon sesame oil
- 1 teaspoon ginger, grated
- 2 cloves garlic, minced
- Cooked brown rice or quinoa

Instructions:

- Heat sesame oil in a pan over medium heat. Add tofu and cook until golden brown on all sides.
- Add garlic and ginger, sauté for 1 minute.
- Add mixed vegetables and stir-fry until just tender (about 5 minutes).
- Stir in soy sauce and cook for another minute.
- Serve over brown rice or quinoa.

3. Baked Chicken Breast with Sweet Potatoes and Green Beans:

Ingredients:

- 2 chicken breasts
- 2 sweet potatoes, diced
- 2 cups green beans, trimmed
- Olive oil
- Salt, pepper, and your choice of herbs (rosemary or thyme work well)

Instructions:

- Preheat the oven to 400°F (200°C).
- Toss sweet potatoes and green beans in olive oil, salt, pepper, and herbs. Spread on a baking sheet.
- Place chicken breasts on the same sheet, season with salt, pepper, and herbs.

- Bake for 25-30 minutes, or until chicken is cooked through and vegetables are tender.

4. Whole Wheat Pasta with Marinara and Vegetables:

Ingredients:

- 8 oz whole wheat pasta
- 1 jar marinara sauce
- 1 zucchini, diced
- 1 cup spinach
- 1/2 cup mushrooms, sliced
- Olive oil
- Grated Parmesan cheese (optional)

Instructions:

- Cook whole wheat pasta according to package instructions. Drain and set aside.

- In a skillet, heat olive oil over medium heat. Sauté mushrooms and zucchini until tender.
- Add spinach and cook until wilted.
- Stir in marinara sauce and heat through.
- Toss cooked pasta with the sauce and serve with grated Parmesan if desired.

5. Chickpea and Spinach Curry:

Ingredients:

- 1 can chickpeas (rinsed and drained)
- 2 cups fresh spinach
- 1 onion, chopped
- 2 garlic cloves, minced
- 1 tablespoon curry powder
- 1 can coconut milk
- Olive oil

- Salt and pepper
- Cooked brown rice or quinoa

Instructions:

- In a pot, heat olive oil over medium heat. Add onion and cook until soft.
- Stir in garlic and curry powder, cooking for 1 minute.
- Add chickpeas and coconut milk, simmer for 10 minutes.
- Stir in spinach until wilted. Season with salt and pepper.
- Serve over brown rice or quinoa.

These dinner recipes are nutritious and flavorful, making them perfect for a healthy meal!

Snacks & Desserts Recipes

Here are some healthy snack and dessert recipes that are easy to make and delicious!

Snacks:

1. Veggie Sticks with Hummus:

Ingredients:

- Carrot sticks, cucumber slices, and bell pepper strips
- 1/2 cup hummus

Instructions:

- Slice vegetables into sticks.
- Serve with hummus for dipping.

2. Greek Yogurt Parfait:

Ingredients:

- 1 cup Greek yogurt

- 1/2 cup mixed berries (fresh or frozen)
- 1 tablespoon honey or maple syrup
- 2 tablespoons granola

Instructions:

- Layer Greek yogurt, berries, honey, and granola in a glass or bowl.
- Repeat layers as desired and enjoy!

3. Apple Slices with Nut Butter:

Ingredients:

- 1 apple, sliced
- 2 tablespoons almond butter or peanut butter

Instructions:

- Slice the apple and spread nut butter on each slice.
- Enjoy as a nutritious snack.

Desserts:

<u>1. Chia Seed Pudding:</u>

Ingredients:

- 1/4 cup chia seeds
- 1 cup almond milk (or any milk)
- 1 tablespoon honey or maple syrup
- Toppings: fresh fruit, nuts, or coconut flakes

Instructions:

- Mix chia seeds, almond milk, and sweetener in a bowl.

- Stir well and let sit for 10 minutes, then stir again.
- Refrigerate for at least 2 hours or overnight.
- Serve with toppings of your choice.

2. Banana Oat Cookies:

Ingredients:

- 2 ripe bananas, mashed
- 1 cup rolled oats
- Optional: 1/4 cup dark chocolate chips or nuts

Instructions:

- Preheat oven to 350°F (175°C).
- In a bowl, mix mashed bananas and oats until combined. Add chocolate chips or nuts if using.

- Drop spoonfuls of the mixture onto a baking sheet lined with parchment paper.
- Bake for 10-12 minutes until golden. Allow to cool before serving.

3. Dark Chocolate-Dipped Strawberries:

Ingredients:

- Fresh strawberries
- 1/2 cup dark chocolate chips

Instructions:

- Melt dark chocolate chips in a microwave-safe bowl, stirring until smooth.
- Dip each strawberry halfway into the melted chocolate and place on parchment paper.

- Let the chocolate harden at room temperature or refrigerate until set.

These snacks and desserts are not only tasty but also nutritious, perfect for satisfying cravings in a healthy way!

CHAPTER THREE
Supplements And Natural Remedies

Here are some common supplements and natural remedies that may help with constipation:

Supplements:

Fiber Supplements:

- **Psyllium husk**: A soluble fiber that can help soften stools and improve bowel regularity.
- **Methylcellulose**: A plant-based fiber that absorbs water and adds bulk to stool.

Probiotics:

• Probiotic supplements can help balance gut bacteria, potentially improving digestive health and promoting regularity.

Magnesium:

- Magnesium supplements can help relax the muscles in the intestines, promoting bowel movements.

Flaxseed Oil:

- Rich in omega-3 fatty acids, flaxseed oil can help lubricate the intestines and improve stool consistency.

Natural Remedies:

Prunes:

- Prunes (dried plums) are well-known for their natural laxative effects due to their high fiber and sorbitol content.

Warm Water with Lemon:

- Drinking warm water with lemon juice in the morning can help stimulate digestion and promote regular bowel movements.

Aloe Vera:

- Aloe vera juice may help soothe the digestive tract and promote bowel regularity, but it should be consumed in moderation due to potential laxative effects.

Peppermint Tea:

- Peppermint can help relax the digestive system and relieve bloating, which may indirectly help with constipation.

Olive Oil:

- Consuming a tablespoon of olive oil on an empty stomach may help lubricate the intestines and promote smoother bowel movements.

Regular Physical Activity:

- Engaging in regular exercise can stimulate the digestive system and help prevent constipation.

Always consult with a healthcare professional before starting any new supplement or remedy, especially if you have underlying health conditions or are taking other medications.

Lifestyle Factors

Lifestyle factors play a significant role in digestive health and can either contribute to or alleviate constipation. Here are some key lifestyle considerations:

• Consuming a high-fiber diet (fruits, vegetables, whole grains, legumes) helps bulk up stool and promotes regular bowel movements. Drinking plenty of water is essential for softening stool and aiding digestion.

• Engaging in regular physical activity (walking, jogging, yoga) helps stimulate bowel function and can alleviate constipation.

• Setting aside time for regular bowel movements, ideally after meals, can help train the body and improve regularity.

- Stress can negatively impact digestive health. Practices like mindfulness, meditation, and deep breathing can help manage stress levels.

- Getting enough restful sleep is important for overall health and can positively influence digestive function.

- Excessive consumption can lead to dehydration, which may contribute to constipation.

- Some medications can cause constipation as a side effect. Discuss any concerns with a healthcare provider.

- Ignoring the urge to have a bowel movement can lead to constipation over time. It's important to respond promptly when the urge arises.

By adopting these lifestyle practices, individuals can enhance their digestive health and reduce the risk of constipation.

Monitoring And Adjusting Your Diet

Monitoring and adjusting your diet can be an effective strategy for managing constipation and improving overall digestive health. Here are some tips on how to do this:

1. Keep a Food Diary:

• **Track Intake**: Record what you eat and drink daily, along with any symptoms of constipation.

• **Identify Patterns**: Look for connections between your diet and digestive issues to identify foods that may contribute to or alleviate constipation.

2. Increase Fiber Gradually:

- **Introduce Fiber Slowly**: If you need to increase your fiber intake, do so gradually to avoid gas and bloating.

- **Aim for Variety**: Include both soluble (oats, beans, fruits) and insoluble (whole grains, nuts, vegetables) fibers for optimal results.

3. Stay Hydrated:

- **Monitor Fluid Intake**: Ensure you're drinking enough water throughout the day, especially as you increase fiber intake.

- **Track Hydration**: Consider keeping a log of your daily water consumption to ensure adequate hydration.

4. Limit Trigger Foods:

• **Identify Problem Foods**: Pay attention to foods that may cause constipation (e.g., processed foods, dairy) and consider reducing or eliminating them.

• **Experiment with Alternatives**: Try substitutes for high-fat or low-fiber foods to see if your symptoms improve.

5. Plan Balanced Meals:

• **Include Whole Foods**: Focus on whole, unprocessed foods that are naturally high in fiber and nutrients.

• **Monitor Portion Sizes**: Overeating can lead to discomfort, so be mindful of portion sizes.

6. Adjust Based on Symptoms:

- **Be Flexible**: If certain foods worsen your constipation, adjust your diet accordingly.

- **Consult a Professional**: Consider working with a registered dietitian for personalized guidance based on your specific needs and symptoms.

7. Incorporate Probiotics:

- **Include Fermented Foods**: Foods like yogurt, kefir, sauerkraut, and kimchi can help support gut health and improve digestion.

By actively monitoring and adjusting your diet, you can make informed choices that support digestive health and alleviate constipation.

Conclusion

Managing constipation involves a holistic approach that includes dietary modifications, lifestyle changes, and mindful practices. Key strategies include:

- **Dietary Adjustments**: Increasing fiber intake through fruits, vegetables, whole grains, and legumes, while staying adequately hydrated, can significantly improve bowel regularity.
- **Physical Activity**: Regular exercise stimulates digestion and helps prevent constipation.
- **Routine and Awareness**: Establishing a regular bowel routine, listening to your body's urges, and maintaining a food diary can help identify patterns and trigger foods.

- **Stress Management**: Implementing stress-reduction techniques can positively impact digestive health.
- **Consultation**: If constipation persists, seeking advice from a healthcare professional or registered dietitian can provide personalized strategies and address any underlying issues.

By adopting these practices, individuals can enhance their digestive health, promote regularity, and improve their overall well-being.

THE END

www.ingramcontent.com/pod-product-compliance
Lightning Source LLC
Chambersburg PA
CBHW030049230526
45471CB00003B/1016